# Alzheimer's Prevention Diet

## A 4-Week Quick Start Meal Plan With Tasty Curated Recipes

mf

copyright © 2021 Jeffrey Winzant

All rights reserved No part of this book may be reproduced, or stored in a retrieval system, or transmitted in any form or by any means, electronic, mechanical, photocopying, recording, or otherwise, without express written permission of the publisher.

# Disclaimer

By reading this disclaimer, you are accepting the terms of the disclaimer in full. If you disagree with this disclaimer, please do not read the guide.

All of the content within this guide is provided for informational and educational purposes only, and should not be accepted as independent medical or other professional advice. The author is not a doctor, physician, nurse, mental health provider, or registered nutritionist/dietician. Therefore, using and reading this guide does not establish any form of a physician-patient relationship.

Always consult with a physician or another qualified health provider with any issues or questions you might have regarding any sort of medical condition. Do not ever disregard any qualified professional medical advice or delay seeking that advice because of anything you have read in this guide. The information in this guide is not intended to be any sort of medical advice and should not be used in lieu of any medical advice by a licensed and qualified medical professional.

The information in this guide has been compiled from a variety of known sources. However, the author cannot attest to or guarantee the accuracy of each source and thus should not be held liable for any errors or omissions.

You acknowledge that the publisher of this guide will not be held liable for any loss or damage of any kind incurred as a result of this guide or the reliance on any information provided within this guide. You acknowledge and agree that you assume all risk and responsibility for any action you undertake in response to the information in this guide.

Using this guide does not guarantee any particular result (e.g., weight loss or a cure). By reading this guide, you acknowledge that there are no guarantees to any specific outcome or results you can expect.

All product names, diet plans, or names used in this guide are for identification purposes only and are the property of their respective owners. The use of these names does not imply endorsement. All other trademarks cited herein are the property of their respective owners.

Where applicable, this guide is not intended to be a substitute for the original work of this diet plan and is, at most, a supplement to the original work for this diet plan and never a direct substitute. This guide is a personal expression of the facts of that diet plan.

Where applicable, persons shown in the cover images are stock photography models and the publisher has obtained the rights to use the images through license agreements with third-party stock image companies.

# Table of Contents

**Introduction**   7
**What Is the Alzheimer's Prevention Diet?**   9
   What is this diet all about?   10
   Weekly Meal Planning   12
   The Top 10 Brain-Healthy Foods   12
   Foods to Avoid   16
**Week 1 Meal Plan**   20
   Week 1 Meal Plan   20
**Sample Recipes for Week 1**   24
   Turmeric Tea   25
   Chia Seed and Strawberry Pudding   26
   Quinoa Lentil Salad   27
   Ikarian Stew with Black-Eyed Peas   29
**Week 2 Meal Plan**   31
   Week 2 Meal Plan   31
**Sample Recipes for Week 2**   34
   Apricot-Glazed Salmon   35
   Vegetable and Tofu Chili Sauté   36
   Fresh Asparagus Salad   38
   Roast Broccoli and Salmon   40
**Week 3 Meal Plan**   42
   Week 3 Meal Plan   43
**Sample Recipes Week 3**   46
   Blueberry Pancakes   47
   Spicy and Sweet Pad Thai   49
   Baked Salmon   51
   Pine Nut Quinoa Bowl   52
**Week 4 Meal Plan**   54
   Week 4 Meal Plan   55

| | |
|---|---:|
| **Sample Recipes for Week 4** | **57** |
|     Strawberry Smoothie | 58 |
|     Balsamic-Glazed Chicken Thighs | 59 |
|     Shrimp Avocado Salad | 60 |
|     Chicken Wrap (Cajun Style) | 62 |
| **Conclusion** | **63** |
| **References and Helpful Links** | **65** |

# Introduction

Alzheimer's Disease (AD) is a progressive and irreversible brain disorder. It slowly destroys thinking skills and memory. Eventually, the patient will lose the ability to carry out simple tasks.

Most symptoms of this illness first appear when one is in their mid-60s. Today, over 5.5 million Americans have dementia caused by AD. It's also the 6th leading cause of death in the United States.

According to Christopher Ochner, a Harvard-trained neurologist, the simplest prevention of the disease is eating properly. However, some people eat nutritious foods, but they still end up having Alzheimer's. So what's the secret?

Healthy eating and following the Alzheimer's diet are the best dietary programs for the prevention of the onset of AD. The diet, particularly, can ease symptoms and improve memory, cognition, and longevity.

Most people don't understand the implications of AD. Until it happens to someone they love, they don't get how serious this disease is. Don't wait till you or your loved one wastes away because of Alzheimer's disease. Alzheimer's diet can improve the life of someone who is now suffering from AD. It's the best all-natural method that can combat Alzheimer's.

In this guide, you'll learn about the following:

- All about the Alzheimer's diet
- Benefits of the diet
- Food to consume and avoid in this diet
- Step-by-step guide in following a weekly meal plan
- Recipes perfect for the Alzheimer's diet

The techniques, as well as the brain-healthy recipes and tips in this book, are based on the results and empirical research of hundreds of studies conducted over the last two decades.

Thanks again for getting this guide. I hope you enjoy it!

# What Is the Alzheimer's Prevention Diet?

Alzheimer's disease, or AD, is a chronic neurodegenerative disease. It usually starts slowly, and it worsens over time. In other words, Alzheimer's is a debilitating disease, which causes irreparable damage to the brain. 60 to 70 percent of dementia cases are due to AD, according to the World Health Organization (WHO).

The causes of this illness are poorly understood. However, studies have proven that good nutrition can improve their symptoms and stop the disease from getting worse. Keeping a healthy weight and eating selected foods can improve language and behavioral problems.

As stated in a 2017 study by Landes Bioscience, good food and nutrition can delay and prevent chronic disability. This is beneficial to the elderly population. Some foods can influence biological and biochemical processes. Bioactive components, including choline, flavonoids, and carotenoids, can preserve and restore healthy brain status.

However, certain cooking procedures can alter the contents of healthy ingredients and cause the loss of healthy nutrients. Thus, the method of cooking must also be considered. The good news is that the Alzheimer's diet is designed to retain the bioactive compounds in ingredients, such as nuts, berries, and leafy vegetables so that one can truly absorb the nutrients from healthy ingredients.

## What is this diet all about?

The AD diet is rich in vitamins and low in saturated fats. It has been revealed that saturated fat or bad fat contributes to the development of heart disease and neurodegenerative diseases. In a Harvard study involving 6,000 women, the people who ate bad fat had the worst thinking ability and memory over time.

Additionally, people who eat meals high in simple carbohydrates, which include mono- and disaccharides, are also at risk of having dementia and AD. Excessive use of beer is also associated with a high risk of AD.

In contrast, caffeine, cocoa, red wine, and tea decrease the risk of having the disease. The AD diet or the mind diet recommends the intake of one glass of wine a day. Wine is one of the top ten brain-healthy foods that help prevent Alzheimer's disease:

- Wine
- Olive oil

- Poultry
- Fish
- Whole grains
- Beans
- Berries
- Leafy vegetables
- Nuts
- Fruits and other vegetables

Vitamin E from fruits and vegetables can slow cognitive decline. Omega 3 fatty acids and B vitamins can slow the rate of cognitive and clinical decline. This is according to several studies conducted in 2013, including the survey of the Institute of Public Health of the United Arab Emirates.

The final scores for CDR sum-of-boxes, global cognition, and verbal delayed recall in the omega-3 and B vitamins group were better than the subjects who were given a normal diet. The effect of B vitamins on cognitive decline was improved when omega-3 fatty acids-rich foods were added to the diet.

When omega-3 levels are higher than normal in the body, B vitamins can slow cognitive decline. In conclusion, it's best to combine foods rich in B vitamins and omega-3 in one meal. The next chapter will explore the best healthy combinations for combating Alzheimer's.

## Weekly Meal Planning

Regular nutritious meals are important for people with Alzheimer's disease. Optimized for brain health, the Alzheimer's diet prevents dementia, protects memory, and prevents loss of brain function.

It encourages the consumption of wine, poultry, beans, fish, healthy oils, whole grains, nuts, berries, and vegetables. Naturally, some of these foodstuffs can be hard to eat, and people crave red meat and other unhealthy foods from time to time.

However, with tasty and creative dishes and a meal plan for each week of the month, preparing nutritious, appetizing meals for a patient with AD won't be a challenge at all.

## The Top 10 Brain-Healthy Foods

Currently, the diet has no set guidelines. It only promotes the proper preparation and consumption of foods from ten nutritious food groups. The patient must also eat less of the five unhealthy foods listed in the succeeding section.

The foods below, on the contrary, contain bioactive compounds and nutrients that promote brain health. They also reduce the formation of amyloid plaques, which destroy connections between neurons.

**Leafy Veggies**

Frequent servings of green and leafy vegetables are recommended. Collards, broccoli, and spinach are packed with vitamins A, C, and K. Two servings per week can help. However, researchers found out that six or more vegetable dishes a week is the best option.

**Other Vegetables**

Eating other vegetables in combination with leafy veggies once a day quenches hunger and cravings for starchy foods. Carrots, beets, and squash provide a lot of nutrients and high calories.

Dietitians recommend eating one veggie salad per day.

**Berries**

Berries are packed with antioxidants that can delay brain aging and improve memory.

Blueberries provide various health benefits. They deliver anthocyanins. Anthocyanins are plant compounds with antioxidant and anti-inflammatory effects.

Antioxidants prevent inflammation, oxidative stress, and other conditions that contribute to neurodegenerative diseases and brain aging.

Also, antioxidants, like lycopene and carotenoids, accumulate in the brain and improve communication and relaying between neurons. They can also delay short-term memory loss.

You can sprinkle berries over breakfast cereals, fruit juices, and desserts.

**Nuts**

As best as you can, provide at least five servings of nuts per week. Also, don't just use one type of nut for your dishes, but try to incorporate several nutritious nuts like walnuts and hazelnuts.

Studies have shown that nuts can improve heart health and brain health. In a 2014 study, nuts, such as almonds and pecan nuts, prevent AD and improve cognition.

Another study also revealed that people who ate at least three servings per week over 2 to 3 years had a sharper memory than those who didn't.

Nutrients, such as vitamin E, antioxidants, and omega-3, are the reason why eating nuts is beneficial for the brain. Vitamin E protects the cell membranes of the neurons from free radical damage. This prevents mental decline. Walnuts, for example, are rich in omega-3 fatty acids, zinc, and vitamin E.

## Healthy Oils

Use olive and coconut oil in cooking vegetables and lean meat. They contain healthy monounsaturated fats and anti-inflammatory properties. As stated in the Journal of Nutrition, Health, and Aging, the people who had been given extra-virgin olive oil as a supplement to their diet were more fluent and performed better in memory tasks than those who had had normal diets.

## Whole Grains

Whole grains, such as barley and brown rice, are jam-packed with nutrients, which include B vitamins, trace minerals, fiber, and protein. A diet that is rich in whole grains can reduce the risk of heart disease, cancer, obesity, AD, and type 2 diabetes.

## Fish

Fishes provide healthy lean meat. Eating fish dishes once a week protects brain function. Choose fatty fish, such as mackerel, tuna, trout, sardines, and salmon, for they contain high amounts of omega-3.

## Beans

Beans must be given regularly to AD patients. Beans are high in protein and fiber, and they are low in fat and calories. As part of the diet, they keep one's mind alert and sharp. It is recommended to consume three servings of beans per week.

Soy products, such as soya milk and soya bread, are alternatives for soybeans when it isn't available.

## Poultry

Eat turkey or chicken at least two times a week. However, fried chicken must not be added to the diet. Meat from two-legged animals is healthier than meat from four-legged animals.

## Wine

Serve one glass of red wine after dinner every day. Red wine has anti-inflammatory properties, and it gets rid of toxins associated with AD. The resveratrol from wine also protects brain cells from damage.

# Foods to Avoid

The AD diet recommends limiting the consumption of the foods below:

## Margarine and Butter

Patients must only intake less than 1 tbsp. of margarine per week. Instead of margarine, butter, or palm oil, use healthy oils as a primary cooking fat. Dietitians also advised dipping wheat bread in extra-virgin olive oil with herbs.

## Cheese

Cheese may be savory, but saturated fat from dairy foods can cause cholesterol build-up and heart diseases, as well as depression and neurodegenerative diseases. One serving per week is okay.

## Red Meat

Red meat, which includes pork, lamb, and beef products, should be eaten three times per week only. Remember that saturated fat from red meat contributes to memory loss.

## Fried Foods

This includes dishes from fast food restaurants and foods coated with marinade high in sodium. Limit consumption of red meat to less than once a month.

## Sweets and Pastries

Candies, doughnuts, cakes, brownies, cookies, and ice cream should be taken in moderation. They contain trans fat and are jam-packed with sugar, including mono- and disaccharides. Patients must also refrain from eating other junk foods, including sodas and instant snacks.

The foods above contain trans fats and saturated fats. These two are associated with numerous diseases, such as AD, hypertension, and heart disease. They affect memory function and increase inflammation.

AD patients often need to maintain weight. The Alzheimer's diet focuses on maintaining overall health, and this includes maintaining a healthy weight. Loss of appetite and muscle mass are major issues for elderly people.

The diet promotes the intake of nutrition-packed foods that encourage eating. You don't need to turn to processed foods or dishes high in artificial flavors to feed your loved one or yourself. Just provide meals high in protein, calories, and healthy oil.

Chicken, turkey, nuts, and eggs can encourage eating on time. High-calorie beverages, such as smoothies, milk, and a protein shake, can greatly contribute to the daily calorie requirement of your patient.

You should start by giving small frequent meals. Three meals a day is sufficient. The patient shouldn't skip breakfast, lunch, and dinner. After week 4, as he or she gets used to the change, you can introduce snacks based on the AD, DASH, and Mediterranean diet.

Salads and soups should be given at least 1-2 times a day. Vegetables, nuts, and fruits are loaded with minerals and vitamins. The said ingredients are the main constituents of salads.

Soups preserve the nutritional value of fresh ingredients. Broth and soups warm and soften the stomach. They are rich in taste, healthy and nutritious, and a good source of fluids.

If the patient has trouble eating, broth and gruel can be given to provide protein to his or her body. Protein is important in maintaining muscle mass, strength, and normal brain function.

Red meat isn't encouraged. On the other hand, seafood and poultry are good sources of protein and have low trans fats. Seafood, including mollusks and fishes, are great sources of Omega-3 and other healthy oils.

# Week 1 Meal Plan

Now you know the key ingredients for the diet and what foods to avoid, it's time to formulate a weekly meal plan. The AD diet is simpler to follow than other diet regimens.

All you have to remember are the following rules: a glass of wine a day should be given to the patient and refrain from serving meals high in saturated and trans fats. To get started, use the sample template for week 1 below.

## Week 1 Meal Plan

### Monday

- Breakfast: Greek yogurt topped with fresh slices of raspberries and sliced almonds
- Lunch: Mediterranean salad with whole wheat pita and grilled chicken
- Dinner: Burrito bowl with guacamole, salsa, grilled chicken, quinoa and lentil salad, black beans, and brown rice

## Tuesday

- Breakfast: Scrambled eggs with French toast
- Lunch: A bowl of blackberries and carrots and a grilled chicken sandwich
- Dinner: Grilled salmon, brown rice, and veggie salad with olive oil dressing

## Wednesday

- Breakfast: Oatmeal with strawberry slices on top and two hard-boiled eggs
- Lunch: Mexican salad with mixed olive oil dressing, grilled chicken, corn, red onion, black beans, and mixed greens
- Dinner: Brown rice and veggie and chicken stir-fry

## Thursday

- Breakfast: Banana and peanut butter Greek yogurt
- Lunch: Black-eyed peas, collard greens, baked trout, and chia seeds, and strawberry pudding
- Dinner: Turkey meatballs whole wheat spaghetti and olive-based veggie salad

## Friday

- Breakfast: Wheat toast topped with avocado slices and onions and sweet peppers omelet
- Lunch: Grilled spicy turkey with grilled veggies on the side

- Dinner: Wheat dinner roll, side salad, baked potatoes, Greek baked chicken

**Saturday**

- Breakfast: Overnight oats topped with strawberry slices
- Lunch: Pinto beans, brown rice, whole wheat tortillas fish tacos
- Dinner: Whole wheat pita chicken gyro and tomato and sea cucumber salad

**Sunday**

- Breakfast: Spinach frittata, peanut butter, apple slices, and turmeric tea
- Lunch: Wheat bread tuna salad sandwich and carrots and celery humus
- Dinner: Brown rice, grilled lentils, and chicken curry

After each dinner, make it a habit to serve one glass of wine to each patient.

Vegetables and whole wheat are both staple foods in the AD diet. Aside from healthy pudding and tea, salads with olive oil dressings are the easiest meals to prepare.

A simple balsamic vinaigrette can serve as an alternative. Just combine three parts of canola oil with one part of balsamic vinegar for your preferred veggies and nuts. Sprinkle a pinch of salt and pepper and half a teaspoon of Dijon mustard. Mix well to soak the vegetables with the seasonings. For more recipes, peruse the next chapter.

# Sample Recipes for Week 1

# Turmeric Tea

**Ingredients:**

- 1/2 tsp. of turmeric
- 1/4 tsp. finely chopped ginger or ginger powder
- 1 cup almond milk
- 1 tsp. honey
- 1 tsp. cinnamon

**Instructions:**

1. Microwave almond milk for 3 minutes.
2. Stir in the ginger, cinnamon, and turmeric.
3. Drizzle honey.
4. Serve and enjoy.

# Chia Seed and Strawberry Pudding

**Ingredients:**

- 1 cup strawberries, thinly sliced
- 3 tbsp. chia seeds
- 1 cup soy beverage, unsweetened and fortified

**Instructions:**

1. To create pudding, combine the soy beverage and chia seeds.
2. Refrigerate the mixture for half an hour. Stir the mixture every 5 minutes to prevent the chia seeds from sticking together.
3. As an alternative, blend the soy beverage and chia seeds in a food processor and let it chill in the refrigerator.
4. Slice strawberries lengthwise.
5. Pour chilled pudding into 2 glasses. Place the strawberry slices on top.
6. Serve and enjoy your pudding.

# Quinoa Lentil Salad

**Ingredients:**

- 2/3 cups dried brown lentils
- 2 cups water
- 1 cup quinoa
- 1 yellow sweet pepper, diced
- 1 shallot, chopped
- 1 bunch arugula, finely chopped
- 2 tsp. Dijon mustard
- 1/4 cup lemon juice
- 1/4 cup extra virgin olive oil
- 1/3 cup crumbled feta cheese
- 1 pinch salt
- 4 tbsp. fresh mint, chopped

**Instructions:**

1. Bring 2 cups of salt water to a boil in a saucepan.
2. Toss veggies into boiling salt water. Lower heat, and cook for 30 minutes.
3. Drain lentils and discard water. Set veggies aside.
4. Boil another batch of saltwater, and cook the quinoa in the pan.
5. In a bowl, mix pepper, salt, mustard, lemon juice, and oil.

6. Place veggies in a larger bowl, and pour the mixture.
7. Sprinkle mint and feta cheese over the salad.
8. Serve and enjoy.

# Ikarian Stew with Black-Eyed Peas

**Ingredients:**

- 2 cups dried black-eyed peas, discard stones and drain and rinse after soaking for an hour
- 2 garlic cloves, minced
- 1 onion, chopped
- 1 fennel bulb, trimmed, halved, and sliced into thin strips
- 4 celery stalks, chopped
- 3 carrots, peeled and chopped
- 1 tomato, diced
- 2 bay leaves
- 3 tbsp. tomato paste
- 1 tsp. salt
- 1/2 cup fresh dill, chopped
- 4 large kale leaves, slivered
- olive oil

**Instructions:**

1. Drain and rinse the peas before proceeding with the recipe.
2. Place the peas, garlic, onion, carrots, fennel, tomato, and celery in the slow cooker. Cover with water.
3. Add bay leaves, salt, and tomato paste.
4. Place the lid and set it to cook on low for 7 hours.

5. Add the dill and kale leaves about 15-20 minutes before the cooking time is done.
6. Leave to cook until the time is over or until the kale is soft.
7. Season with pepper and salt according to desired taste.
8. Upon serving, drizzle with olive oil and enjoy while hot.

# Week 2 Meal Plan

Meal planning for the Alzheimer's diet is easy and simple. You only need to concentrate on the ten food groups listed in Chapter 2 to prepare nutritious meals. Also, limit serving junk foods and dishes that are high in cholesterol, refined sugars, bad fat, and sodium.

The meal plan below is approved by dietitians and neurologists. Dr. Christopher Ochner, a Columbia alumnus and nutritionist, formulated an eating itinerary for the elderly. This weekly meal plan is based on Dr. Ochner's research.

## Week 2 Meal Plan

**Monday**

- Breakfast: Chocolate overnight oats with strawberry vanilla compote
- Lunch: Lemonade avocado pesto and zucchini noodles soup
- Dinner: Honey mustard chicken salad, rainbow rotisserie, and a glass of wine

## Tuesday

- Breakfast: No ham scrambled green eggs and 1 slice of gluten-free toast
- Lunch: Leftover chicken salad plus 2 slices of watermelon
- Dinner: 4 apple slices with cinnamon, crunchy lentil tacos, and a glass of wine

## Wednesday

- Breakfast: Sugar-free Greek yogurt and oatmeal chia crisp
- Lunch: Quinoa lentil salad, lemon and almonds vinaigrette, and 3 cherry tomatoes
- Dinner: Pan-seared salmon, steamed broccoli with olive oil, and forbidden rice

## Thursday

- Breakfast: Fresh asparagus salad and a slice of wheat bread
- Lunch: Apricot glazed salmon and turmeric tea
- Dinner: Vegetable and tofu chili sauté

## Friday

- Breakfast: Walnut-blueberry pancakes and chocolate blueberry smoothie
- Lunch: Black-eyed peas longevity stew
- Dinner: Tuscan baked beans with basil and kale

**Saturday**

- Breakfast: Buckwheat flapjacks
- Lunch: Greek yogurt chicken ties with steamed olives and artichokes
- Dinner: Orange-cranberry turkey and potato salad

**Sunday**

- Breakfast: Sweet corn, bell peppers, and chicken zucchini basil frittata
- Lunch: Pecan-crusted chicken stuffed with asparagus
- Dinner: Three ways mussels and apple slices

# Sample Recipes for Week 2

# Apricot-Glazed Salmon

**Ingredients:**

- 1-1/3 pounds wild salmon filets
- 1/4 tsp. of crushed black pepper*
- 1 tbsp. virgin olive oil
- 1/2 cup of sodium-free vegetable broth
- 1 tbsp. Dijon mustard
- 1/3 cup of 100% apricot fruit spread
- 1 tsp. minced garlic

**Instructions:**

1. Preheat the grill over medium heat.
2. Pat salmon dry with a paper towel and cut it into four slices.
3. Season the skinless side with black pepper.
4. Wrap each piece with aluminum foil, with the skin side down. Fold the foil around the salmon securely to prevent oil from leaking.
5. In a bowl, combine the remaining ingredients.
6. Pour the mixture over the salmon slices.
7. Grill salmon for ten minutes.
8. Once cooked, allow the grilled filet to cool down before unwrapping.
9. Plate nicely and garnish with your favorite herbs before serving.

*black pepper may be substituted with white pepper

## Vegetable and Tofu Chili Sauté

**Ingredients:**

- 1 onion, chopped
- 1 stalk, diced
- 1 carrot, diced
- 1/2 chili pepper, minced
- 2 garlic cloves, minced
- 1 green pepper, finely sliced
- 1 cup finely diced tofu
- 6 tsp. avocado oil
- 1 tbsp. brown sugar
- 1 tsp. ground cumin
- 2 cups red beans
- 1-1/2 cups of diced tomatoes
- 1 pinch salt
- 1 pinch ground pepper
- 1/3 cup grated cheddar cheese
- 4 tsp. fresh cilantro

**Instructions:**

1. Warm serving plates in the microwave to keep the salad warm.
2. Heat the avocado oil in a saucepan. Sauté garlic and onion for 2 minutes.
3. Toss in the vegetables. Cook for 4 minutes, stirring occasionally.

4. Pour brown sugar and toss in minced cumin and chili pepper. Cook for another minute.
5. Add in tofu and cook for 8-10 minutes.
6. Drain red and green beans and add to the saucepan. Stir well.
7. Toss in diced tomatoes and pour 1/8 cup of water, mix well. Cook for 10 minutes over low heat.
8. Add pepper and salt to taste. Pour the contents into the heated dishes.
9. Sprinkle cheddar and cilantro leaves when serving.

# Fresh Asparagus Salad

**Ingredients:**

- 1/3 cup of hazelnuts
- 4 cups arugula
- 1 tsp. ground pepper
- 4 tsp. lemon juice
- 2 tbsp. sea salt
- virgin olive oil
- 2 lbs. asparagus

**Instructions:**

1. Preheat the oven to 400°F.
2. Place hazelnuts on a baking tray with parchment paper. Place in the oven for 7 minutes.
3. Transfer hazelnuts to a plate. Optionally, to remove the skins, wrap the nuts in a towel and rub them vigorously.
4. Chop hazelnuts coarsely.
5. Remove the hard ends of the asparagus.
6. Place the stalks on the baking sheet you've used for the hazelnuts. Sprinkle 1 tbsp. olive oil and 1/2 tsp. of salt.
7. Bake for 8 minutes.
8. In a mixing bowl, combine pepper, salt, olive oil, and lemon juice. Mix well.

9. Place the arugula in a medium bowl. Drizzle ½ of the dressing over the veggies. Toss until everything is well coated.
10. Place arugula onto a platter.
11. Arrange asparagus on top. Sprinkle peeled hazelnuts on top.

# Roast Broccoli and Salmon

**Ingredients:**

- 1 bunch broccoli, cut into florets
- 4 tbsp. canola oil, divided
- salt
- pepper
- 4 pcs. salmon filets, skins removed
- 1 pc. jalapeño or red Fresno chile, seeds removed, sliced into thin rings
- 2 tbsp. rice vinegar, unseasoned
- 2 tbsp. capers, drained

**Instructions:**

1. Preheat the oven to 400° F.
2. On a large, rimmed baking sheet, put the broccoli florets and toss in 2 tablespoons of the canola oil. Season with salt and pepper.
3. Roast the florets in the oven for 12 or 15 minutes. Toss occasionally.
4. Remove from the oven when the florets are crisp-tender and browned.
5. Gently rub the filets with 1 tablespoon of the canola oil. Season the salmon with salt and pepper.
6. Put the salmon in the middle of the baking sheet.

7. Move the florets to the sides of the baking sheet. Roast the filet for 10 to 15 minutes or until the filets turn opaque throughout.
8. In a small bowl, combine the vinegar, chile rings, and a pinch of salt.
9. Let the mixture sit for about 10 minutes so that the chile rings become somewhat softened,
10. Add the capers and the remaining tablespoon of canola oil. Add salt and pepper to taste.
11. Drizzle chile vinaigrette over the roasted broccoli and salmon just before serving.

# Week 3 Meal Plan

Reducing pounds and waist circumference are some of the primary purposes of most diet regimens. Similar to other diet plans, the Alzheimer's diet also promotes cholesterol reduction rather than maintaining brain health.

For people who have passed the age of 40, the AD diet is already recommended. Alzheimer's disease often starts in old age. However, there are cases of early onset wherein individuals between the ages of 40 to 50 exhibit symptoms of the disease.

Why does this happen? According to researchers, an unhealthy diet contributes to the early onset of AD. So whether you're caring for patients with AD or you want to preserve your brain health, eating the right foods is necessary.

For week 3, you can start the day with the classic blueberry pancakes and end it with a healthy low-fat butter chicken. For the sides, a baba ghanoush and coconut and ginger ice cream will satisfy your cravings.

# Week 3 Meal Plan

**Monday**

- Breakfast: Strawberry-banana smoothie
- Lunch: Kale salad with Caesar dressing and banana ghanoush
- Dinner: Quinoa and ground turkey chili and coconut and ginger ice cream

**Tuesday**

- Breakfast: a slice of wheat toast and veggie breakfast frittata
- Lunch: a whole wheat bread and tuna salad sandwich
- Dinner: Roasted broccoli and pecan-crusted chicken

**Wednesday**

- Breakfast: Walnut-blueberry pancake
- Lunch: Chicken (grilled) sandwich on wheat bread with hummus and celery
- Dinner: A whole wheat dinner roll, cabbage salad, and roasted turkey

**Thursday**

- Breakfast: 15 almonds and Greek yogurt with blueberries or raspberries
- Lunch: Flavored brown rice with peas and sliced tomatoes and spinach and kale salad with chickpeas,

- tomatoes, mushrooms, bell peppers, carrots, and olive oil dressing
- Dinner: balsamic vinaigrette, roasted broccoli, and whole wheat pasta with marinara sauce and chicken strips

**Friday**

- Breakfast: Oatmeal with almonds and blueberries
- Lunch: 1/2 pita, grilled chicken, and kale salad with tomatoes, feta cheese, olive oil dressing, and chickpeas
- Dinner: Baked salmon with Brussels sprouts and broccoli, quinoa lentil salad, and a glass of wine

**Saturday**

- Breakfast: Whole wheat bagel sandwich, a scrambled egg, and a blueberry pancake
- Lunch: Turkey sandwich on wheat bread with baby carrots, hummus, lettuce, and tomato slices
- Dinner: Vegetables stir fry and quinoa salad with olive oil dressing

**Sunday**

- Breakfast: Avocado slices, banana smoothie, and whole wheat egg sandwich
- Lunch: Caesar salad and spinach salad with olive oil dressing, raspberries, chia seeds, almonds, and strawberries

- Dinner: Baked salmon, grilled trout, sautéed spinach, and 1/2 cup of brown rice

# Sample Recipes Week 3

# Blueberry Pancakes

**Ingredients:**

- 3 omega-3 fresh eggs
- 1 tsp. cinnamon
- 1/2 cup of arrowroot powder
- 1/4 cup of coconut oil
- 1/4 cup walnuts, roughly chopped
- 1 pinch sea salt
- 1/2 tsp. baking soda
- 1/2 tsp. yeast
- 1/2 cup coconut flour
- 1 tsp. vanilla extract
- 1/2 tbsp. lemon juice
- 1-pint blueberries

**Instructions:**

1. Whisk 3 eggs. Pour vanilla, lemon juice, and almond milk. Mix well.
2. In another bowl, combine arrowroot, salt, yeast, baking powder, cinnamon, and coconut flour. Add wet mixture to this mixture while whisking continuously.
3. Fold in the chopped walnuts.
4. Grease a saucepan over medium heat with coconut oil.
5. Once the oil is hot, scoop the mixture with a ladle, and pour the pancakes into the saucepan. Cook until

bubbles form. Repeat this step until the batter is consumed.
6. For the sauce, simmer blueberries in another saucepan.
7. Add 4 tsp. of water. Simmer for 10 minutes.
8. Pour the sauce over a stack of pancakes and serve.

# Spicy and Sweet Pad Thai

**Ingredients:**

- 1 tbsp. peanut oil
- 2 garlic cloves, finely minced
- 1 sweet red pepper, seeded and minced
- 2 tbsp. fresh cilantro leaves
- 1/2 cup of shredded carrots
- 1/2 cup chopped peanuts
- 1 pinch ground red pepper
- 1 tbsp. honey
- 1/4 cup soy sauce
- 1/4 cup lemon extract or lime juice
- 1 package Thai rice noodles
- 1 package tofu, cubed
- 1/2 cup of sliced mushrooms

**Instructions:**

1. In a saucepan, heat oil over medium heat. Toss in tofu, mushrooms, peppers, and garlic. Cook until the veggies soften.
2. Boil noodles for 15-20 minutes.
3. In a bowl, combine crushed red pepper, honey, soy sauce, and lime juice.
4. Pour mixture over cooked veggies. Mix while simmering. Remove the pan from the heat after 5 minutes.

5. Divide the cooked noodles into 4-5 servings. Top each bowl with cilantro, carrots, and peanuts. Pour broth into each bowl.
6. Serve and enjoy while hot.

# Baked Salmon

## Ingredients:

- 2 salmon fillets
- 6 cups of fresh spinach
- 2 tsp. coconut oil
- 1/4 tsp. garlic powder
- 1/4 tsp. turmeric
- 3 large cloves of garlic
- lemon juice
- salt
- pepper

## Instructions:

1. Preheat the oven to 400°F.
2. Line a baking dish with parchment paper.
3. Marinate salmon fillets in lemon juice, coconut oil, garlic powder, turmeric, salt, and pepper.
4. Let it sit for a few minutes. This may also be done the night before to help the juices and flavor get into the salmon.
5. Once the oven is ready, bake salmon for 15 minutes.
6. Cook some of the garlic in a pan with coconut oil.
7. Add spinach and cook until ready. Season with salt and pepper to taste.
8. Take salmon out of the oven and put spinach beside it.
9. Serve and enjoy.

# Pine Nut Quinoa Bowl

**Ingredients:**

- 1 cup dry white quinoa

Marinara sauce:

- 1-1/4 tbsp. agave nectar
- 1/4 cup extra-virgin olive oil, preferably cold-pressed
- 2 cups sun-dried tomatoes, water-soaked for a couple of hours
- 2 tbsp. lemon juice
- 1 cup soaking water used for tomatoes
- 1/2 yellow onion, chopped
- 2 large heirloom or Roma tomatoes, diced
- 1 handful fresh basil leaves, reserve some for garnish
- 3-4 garlic cloves, crushed
- 1 tsp. sea salt
- 2 tsp. dried oregano
- 1/4 cup pine nuts, reserve some for garnish
- a pinch of hot pepper flakes

**Instructions:**

To cook the quinoa:

1. Wash quinoa.
2. Boil quinoa with 2 cups of filtered water in a medium saucepan.
3. Reduce heat to low and let it simmer.

4. Cover and cook for about 15 to 20 minutes. The quinoa must be tender and fluffy and have absorbed all the water.

To make the marinara sauce:

1. Put all the marinara sauce ingredients in a high-speed blender.
2. Blend everything for about 30-45 seconds, or until smooth. Mix with a tamper in between to help with the blending.
3. Optional: To thin out the sauce, use the water you used to soak the tomatoes and pour it into the blender.
4. Optional: Set the sauce to simmer at a low temperature in a medium saucepan for 25 to 30 minutes.
5. Upon serving, pour a spoonful of the marinara sauce over the cooked quinoa.
6. Top with pine nuts and fresh basil leaves.
7. Serve immediately.

# Week 4 Meal Plan

The Alzheimer's diet is a combination of the Mediterranean diet and the DASH diet. It provides all of the benefits that the two have to offer. The primary health benefits of the former are increasing longevity and preventing AD, Parkinson's disease, heart diseases, and stroke; the DASH diet improves bone strength and increases calcium intake.

The AD diet, which reduces the risk of many illnesses in old age, especially Alzheimer's, has also been associated with preventing cancer and improving heart health. According to Rosie Schwartz, an author, dietitian, and cancer researcher, the Alzheimer's diet and the eating patterns it promotes are beneficial for the entire body.

In week 4, the patient's body has already adapted to the eating regimen. He or she may exhibit increased awareness and cognitive responses. Somatic symptoms, such as diarrhea, vomiting, and salivation, might have also been reduced in the past weeks. By this time, loss of appetite isn't a problem anymore.

Without further ado, here is the meal plan for week 4:

# Week 4 Meal Plan

**Monday**

- Breakfast: Sugar-free sesame cookies and black chocolate pudding with raspberries
- Lunch: Greek chicken gyro salad, Italian chicken wrap, and avocado Caprese wrap
- Dinner: Chicken Caprese sandwich, minestrone, and pan-seared citrus shrimp

**Tuesday**

- Breakfast: Supercharged trail mix
- Lunch: Grilled balsamic chicken and olive tapenade
- Dinner: Mussels three ways and turkey and kale meatball soup

**Wednesday**

- Breakfast: Egg Caprese breakfast cups and mini frittatas
- Lunch: Walnut-crusted salmon fillets and roasted chickpeas
- Dinner: Zucchini and linguine noodles with shrimp

**Thursday**

- Breakfast: Asparagus and mushroom frittatas with goat cheese

- Lunch: Greek chicken gyros and tzatziki sauce on the side
- Dinner: Shaved parmesan and arugula salad and veggie egg casserole

**Friday**

- Breakfast: Caprese avocado toast and a few slices of blueberry pie
- Lunch: White bean and Tuscan tuna salad and turkey sandwich with egg and tomato slices
- Dinner: Citrus black-cod with ginger and Pecan wild rice

**Saturday**

- Breakfast: Apple pie, balsamic vinaigrette, and strawberry smoothie
- Lunch: Chicken Caprese sandwich and Greek pasta salad with artichoke hearts and cucumbers
- Dinner: Avocado and citrus shrimp salad, butter chicken, and ½ cup of brown rice

**Sunday**

- Breakfast: Slow-cooker egg casserole and turmeric tea
- Lunch: Couscous with feta cheese and sun-dried tomato and vegetable bowl
- Dinner: Pesto shrimp and arugula salad and Greek chicken marinade

# Sample Recipes for Week 4

# Strawberry Smoothie

**Ingredients:**

- strawberries, 10pcs.
- banana slices
- orange juice, around 100 ml

**Instructions:**

1. Put all the ingredients in a blender.
2. Grind them until smooth.
3. Put it in a glass.

# Balsamic-Glazed Chicken Thighs

**Ingredients:**

- 1 tsp. garlic powder
- 1 tsp. dried basil
- 1/2 tsp. salt
- 1/2 tsp. pepper
- 2 tsp. dehydrated onion
- 4 garlic cloves, minced
- 1 tbsp. extra-virgin olive oil
- 1/2 cup balsamic vinegar, divide equally
- 8 chicken thighs, boneless and skinless
- fresh chopped parsley, for garnish

**Instructions:**

1. In a small bowl, combine the onion, basil, garlic powder, salt, and pepper.
2. Spread the mixture over the chicken on both sides. Set aside.
3. Pour olive oil into the crockpot and add garlic.
4. Pour in half of the balsamic vinegar.
5. Place chicken on top.
6. Gently pour the remaining balsamic vinegar over the chicken.
7. Cover and cook on high for 3 hours.
8. Sprinkle fresh parsley on top to serve.

# Shrimp Avocado Salad

**Ingredients:**

Salad:

- 1/2 lb. large shrimp, peeled
- 2 sweet corn ears, removed from the cob
- 4 cups Romaine lettuce, chopped
- 3 strips of bacon, diced
- 1 avocado, peeled, pitted and diced
- Optional: 1/3 cup Fontina cheese, grated

Buttermilk pesto dressing:

- 1/2 cup buttermilk
- 1/4 cup pesto, homemade or store-bought
- 1/2 cup mayo or Greek yogurt
- 1 tbsp. lemon juice
- 1 small shallot, minced
- salt
- pepper

**Instructions:**

1. Over high heat, place a skillet.
2. Put in the corn kernels when the skillet heats up.
3. Allow to dry roast while stirring occasionally. Cook until the edges start to caramelize and turn brown, or for about 6-8 minutes.
4. Place the roasted corn on a plate and set aside.

5. Lower the heat to medium-high. Fry the bacon using the same skillet, for about 6 minutes, until crispy.
6. Transfer the bacon to a plate.
7. Saute the shrimp in the same skillet until they are cooked.
8. In a bowl, toss the lettuce, corn, avocado, bacon, and shrimp.
9. Whisk all the ingredients together until blended.
10. Season with salt and pepper.

# Chicken Wrap (Cajun Style)

**Ingredients:**

- keto tortilla
- avocado, half will do, chopped
- cajun chicken
- tomato, chopped
- yogurt, preferably plain or organic, to taste
- lettuce, chopped
- cucumber, chopped
- pepper, to taste
- sea salt, to taste

**Instructions:**

1. Except for the tortilla, toss all the ingredients for the salad in a bowl.
2. Heat up the tortilla in the microwave for 15 seconds, then plate it nicely.
3. Gently transfer the salad mix to the center of the tortilla. Once done, fold both sides nicely, similar to how a burrito is wrapped.
4. Slice and enjoy eating.

# Conclusion

Alzheimer's disease is a challenging illness. However, with the right diet and care, one can combat its debilitating symptoms.

Eating the right kinds of foods and preparing them in the right way are the secrets to Alzheimer's diet. High-quality lean meat, leafy vegetables, and whole grains must be the staple food of people with AD.

Nuts, healthy oils, and fruits must be consumed in moderation, while the intake of food high in sodium, bad fats, and refined sugars must be minimized. These include processed food, cakes, muffins, and fried meat.

Legumes, beans, fruit juices, teas, cocoa, and turmeric can serve as supplements and ingredients for side dishes and snacks. Just remember the 10 food groups and what to avoid in creating weekly meal plans, and you are ready to combat Alzheimer's.

Again, thank you for getting this guide!

If you found this guide helpful, please take the time to share your thoughts and post a review. It'd be greatly appreciated!

Thank you and good luck!

# References and Helpful Links

Avoiding Alzheimers: Adjusting your diet to avoid the disease. (n.d.). Retrieved December 16, 2022, from https://www.cbsnews.com/pittsburgh/news/avoiding-alzheimers-adjusting-your-diet-to-avoid-the-disease/.

Can diet prevent Alzheimer's? | Alzheimer's organization. (n.d.). Alzheimersorg. Retrieved December 16, 2022, from https://www.alzheimersorganization.org/diet-and-alzheimers.

Food and eating. Alzheimer's Disease and Dementia. (n.d.). Retrieved December 16, 2022, from https://www.alz.org/help-support/caregiving/daily-care/food-eating.

Luchsinger, J. A., Noble, J. M., & Scarmeas, N. (2007). Diet and Alzheimer's disease. Current Neurology and Neuroscience Reports, 7(5), 366–372. https://doi.org/10.1007/s11910-007-0057-8.

MD, A. E. B. (2020, May 8). What to eat to reduce your risk of Alzheimer's disease. Harvard Health. https://www.health.harvard.edu/blog/what-to-eat-to-reduce-your-risk-of-alzheimers-disease-2020050819774.

Nutrition and dementia: Foods that may induce memory loss & increase Alzheimer's. (n.d.). Alzheimers.Net. Retrieved December 16, 2022, from https://www.alzheimers.net/foods-that-induce-memory-loss.

What do we know about diet and prevention of Alzheimer's disease? (n.d.). National Institute on Aging. Retrieved December 16, 2022, from https://www.nia.nih.gov/health/what-do-we-know-about-diet-and-prevention-alzheimers-disease.

Yusufov, M., Weyandt, L. L., & Piryatinsky, I. (2017). Alzheimer's disease and diet: A systematic review. The International Journal of Neuroscience, 127(2), 161–175. https://doi.org/10.3109/00207454.2016.1155572.

www.ingramcontent.com/pod-product-compliance
Lightning Source LLC
LaVergne TN
LVHW012036060526
838201LV00061B/4638